ADHD Workbook

The Practical Guide for Parents & School Teachers for

Managing ADHD in Kids and Making them Better

Seor Janice

ISBN: 978-1-63750-176-4

Table of Contents

Introduction

Have you read several books on managing ADHD in children, but despite countless efforts to help your child cope and comprehend better in school by paying attention to instructions and detail information, you're still struggling with everyday issues like homework, chores, getting him or her concentrate when been talked to, and simply getting along without pushback and power struggles?

What if you could work with your child, motivating and engage your kids in the process, to create positive change once and for all?

For millions of kids who live with ADHD, feelings of loneliness, frustration, and helplessness are all too common. This book is designed for parents and teachers to help kids with ADHD develop essential skills for managing their ADHD symptoms, while also providing a powerful message of hope and encouragement for their future.

This book is to help kids reframe the way they think about their ADHD issue, and discover that they have special talents that are unique to them. With fun activities that engage their busy minds, This book offers parents, teachers a better understanding of kids with ADHD, their ADHD, and the simple things they can do to feel more confident and in control.

Chapter 1

What to know about ADHD

Attention Deficit Hyperactivity Disorder, often called ADHD, affects an incredible number of children and frequently continues into adulthood. Analysis usually happens through the preschooler years, but it can occur earlier when the kid grows to be a toddler.

Children with ADHD frequently have trouble paying attention, plus they may showcase hyperactive and impulsive behaviours. These features make a difference in the child's interactions with family, friends, and instructors.

In America, there is certainly concern that specific amounts of growing children are getting this diagnosis while some may be taking medication prematurely.

Others claim, on the other hand, an early medical diagnosis can result in far better treatment.

At what age does ADHD begin, and can infants and toddlers have symptoms? As of this early stage, will there be any way to take care of ADHD?

Small children can have ADHD, but there are no guidelines designed for this generation.

The Centers for Disease Control and Avoidance (CDC) have reported that, in 2016, around 6.1 million children age groups 2-17 in the U.S. experienced a medical diagnosis of ADHD. This data included around 388,000 children of ages 2-5 years.

Before 2011, the American Academy of Pediatrics (AAP) only had guidelines for diagnosing ADHD in children ages 6-12 years.

In 2011, they extended their guidelines to add preschoolers and adolescents, widening the number to included age 4-18 years.

Some children get a diagnosis before the age of 4. However, there are no medical guidelines for analysis at this age group.

Symptoms of ADHD in Kids

It could be hard to note the symptoms of ADHD in children younger than four years. A brief attention period, impulsivity, tantrums, and high degrees of activity are standard during certain phases of development. Many children feel the "awful twos," rather than have ADHD.

Children who are extremely active and also have a great deal of energy, however, not ADHD, can usually concentrate when necessary for stories or even look over picture books. Also, they are in a position to put play toys away or sit and execute a puzzle, for example.

Children with ADHD tend to be struggling to do these exact things. They could show extreme behavior that disrupts activities and relationships. For an analysis of ADHD, a kid must show these manners for at least six months in several environments, such as at home with nursery school.

Small children with ADHD may:

- Be restless.

- Run around, climb, and join everything.

- Be constantly "on the run," as though they may be "driven with a motor."

- Talk non-stop.

- Struggle to concentrate or pay attention for long.

- Think it is hard to stay down, take naps, and sit down for meals.

However, some children with ADHD may focus well on things that interest them, such as particular play toys.

If a mother or father or caregiver thinks that their toddler is displaying behavior that is excessive and intense. If this behavior impacts family life and occurs frequently, they need to consult with their child's doctor for an assessment.

What are the first indicators of ADHD?

Recommendations for diagnosing ADHD do not cover children's age range three (3) years or younger.

However, there is certainly evidence that doctors are

diagnosing ADHD in small children.

Factors that could cause a health care provider to think ADHD as of this age include:

Genetic factors

- if the mom used drugs or alcohol during pregnancy.

- If the mom smoked during pregnancy.

- If the mom was subjected to environmental toxins during pregnancy.

- Preterm delivery or low delivery weight.

- Central nervous system problems at critical occasions in development.

- A delay in motion development, conversation, and language.

- behavioral difficulties.

- Family background of ADHD.

The 2010-2011 Countrywide Study of Children's Health in the U.S. discovered that around 194,000 children age groups 2-5 got diagnosed with ADHD throughout the year.

Just how do Doctors Diagnose ADHD?

To be able to diagnose ADHD in an older child, a health care provider may:

- Have Behavior therapy who can study new means of doing things.

- A health care provider or other experts will observe well the kid can do things such as following instructions.

- Execute a medical examination.

- Take a look at personal and family medical histories.

- Consider school records.

- Ask family, educators, babysitters, and instructors to complete a questionnaire.

- Compare symptoms and behavior to ADHD requirements and ranking scales.

To diagnose ADHD in teenagers and adults, a health care provider will also observe and note characteristics, such as:

- Lack of focus on detail when executing tasks.

- Difficulty staying centered on tasks.

- Appearing never to pay attention when spoken to.

- Not following instructions.

- Difficulty organizing chores.

- Often losing things and forgetting to do something.

- Fidgeting rather than having the ability to stay seated.

- Working or climbing in inappropriate places.

- Excessive talk.

- Inability to take action quietly.

- Difficulty looking forward to their turn.

How about diagnosing infants?

For infants, it could be challenging to learn if they would meet these requirements.

Sometimes, a problem with development, like a vocabulary delay, can lead to a wrong medical diagnosis of ADHD.

Other medical ailments can cause comparable symptoms, including:

- A brain injury.

- Learning or vocabulary problems.

- Feeling disorders, including major depression and anxiety.

- Other psychiatric or neurodevelopmental disorders.

- Seizure disorders.

- Sleep problems.

- Thyroid problems.

- Eyesight or hearing problems.

Preschool-age children or infants who show symptoms of ADHD should visit a specialist for an assessment. Another specialist may be considered a conversation pathologist, developmental pediatrician, psychologist, or psychiatrist. They can help your physician make a precise diagnosis.

Treatment for ADHD

You can find guidelines for treating ADHD in children ages four years and older, but there are no guidelines for treating ADHD in toddlers.

In children older, like 4-5 years, a health care provider might recommend:

Behavioral therapy: A parent or teacher could handle this by following instructions and guidelines.

Medication: If symptoms do not improve with behavioral therapy, and mainly if they are average to severe, a health care provider may recommend methylphenidate hydrochloride (Ritalin) and other stimulant medications.

The physician will monitor the dose and change it out, if required, to ensure that the kid experiences the utmost benefit and the fewest possible side effects.

It's essential to notice that the U.S. Food and Medication Administration (FDA) has never approved the utilization of this medication in children under six years old, credited to too little evidence that it's safe or effective.

The FDA remembers that stimulant medications can have side effects, including slowing a child's growth. Early treatment for toddlers; An educational assessment; Behavior therapy can train new means of nearing problems and communication.

The CDC recommends training for parents and behavior therapy for small children. As an initial step, they state that behavior therapy:

- ✓ Shows parents ways to control their child's behavior.

- ✓ Appears to work well as medication in small children.

- ✓ Prevents the medial side effects that may appear with medication.

The therapist will continue to work with the kid to help them learn:

- ✓ New means of behavior that do not cause problems.

- ✓ Modern methods of expressing themselves.

When the kid is old enough to start kindergarten or school, the parents or caregiver should ask the institution about the probability of educational support.

What about medication?

In 2014, a CDC official presented a written report, stating that over 10,000 toddlers aged 2-3 years may be getting medication for ADHD with methods that do not meet up with the established guidelines in the U.S.

The mental health watchdog Citizens Commission on Human Rights has gathered data suggesting that the number of toddlers getting treatment for ADHD and other psychological medical issues in the U.S. may be more significant than this.

They state that as well as the 10,000 toddlers getting ADHD medication:

- ✓ 318,997 are being administered anti-anxiety drugs

- ✓ 46,102 are being given antidepressants

- ✓ 3,760 are getting antipsychotics

They also discovered that among babies aged 12 months or younger:

- ✓ 249,669 are being given antianxiety medications

- ✓ 24,406 are being administered antidepressants

- ✓ 1,422 are getting drugs for ADHD

✓ 654 are taking antipsychotics

The figures above indicate that very young children may be overmedicated.

A couple of no guidelines for treating toddlers or babies with ADHD. However, recommendations for slightly teenagers suggest attempting behavioral therapy before using medication.

Furthermore, one study reviews that almost 50 percent of toddler individuals aged under three (3) and getting psychotropic medications weren't monitored frequently every three months.

This shows that toddlers and babies may be taking ADHD medications for six months at the same time without doctors looking into the effects.

The AAP asks doctors to weigh the potential risks of administering ADHD medication to babies and toddlers against the harm of delaying analysis and treatment.

Chapter 2

Indicators of ADHD

All kids sometimes struggle to give attention, listen and follow directions, sit down still, or wait around for their turn. But also for kids with ADHD, the challenges are more laborious and happen more regularly.

Kids with ADHD may have indications in one, two, or all three of the categories:

Inattentive: Kids who are inattentive (easily distracted) have trouble concentrating their attention, focusing, and remaining on task. They might not pay attention thoroughly to directions, may miss important details, and might not finish what they start. They could daydream or dawdle too much. They could appear absent-minded or forgetful, and lose tabs on their things.

Hyperactive: Hyperactive Kids are fidgety, restless, and easily uninterested. They could have trouble seated still or keeping silent when needed. They could hurry through things and make careless errors. They could climb, leap, or rough house when they shouldn't. Without meaning to, they could act with techniques that disrupt others.

Impulsive: Kids who are spontaneous work prematurely before thinking. They often interrupt, might drive or grab, and discover it's hard to hold back. They could do things without requesting authorization, take things that are not theirs, or action with dangerous techniques. They could have psychological reactions that appear too extreme for the problem.

Sometimes parents and instructors notice symptoms of ADHD whenever a child is very young. But it's normal for little kids to be distractible, restless, impatient, or impulsive; these exact things don't always imply that a kid has ADHD.

Attention, activity, and self-control develop over time as children grow. Kids learn these skills with help from parents and educators. However, many kids do not get far better at getting attended to, settling down, hearing, or waiting around. When these exact things continue and start to cause problems in school, home, and with friends, it might be ADHD.

How is ADHD Diagnosed?

If you believe your son or daughter has ADHD, schedule an appointment with your son or daughter's doctor. He/she will give your son or daughter a check-up, including eyesight and hearing, to make sure another thing isn't leading to the symptoms. The physician can send you to a kid psychologist or psychiatrist if needed.

To diagnose ADHD, doctors begin by asking in regards to a child's health, behavior, and activity. They talk to parents and kids about the things they have observed. Your physician might request you to complete checklists about your son or daughter's behavior and may require you to give your son or daughter's instructor a list too.

After gathering these details, doctors diagnose ADHD, whether it's clear that:

- A child's distractibility, hyperactivity, or impulsivity exceed what's usually of their age.

- The behaviors have been taking place because the child was young.

- Distractibility, hyperactivity, and impulsivity

impact the kid in school and at home.

- A health check demonstrates another health or learning concern isn't leading to the problems.

- Many kids with ADHD likewise have learning problems, oppositional and defiant actions, or mood and anxiety problems; doctors usually treat these combined with the ADHD.

How is ADHD Treated?

Treatment for ADHD usually includes:

Medication: This activates the brain's capability to give attention, decelerate, and use more self-control.

Behavior therapy: Therapists can help kids develop the sociable, psychological, and planning skills that are lagging with ADHD.

Parental training: Through training, parents learn the best ways to react to behavior problems that are part of ADHD.

School support: Educators can help kids with ADHD prosper and enjoy school more.

The proper treatment helps ADHD improve. Parents and instructors can teach more youthful kids to grasp, controlling their attention, behavior, and feelings. As they get older, kids should figure out how to enhance their concentration and self-control.

When ADHD is not treated, it could be hard for kids to achieve success. This may lead to low self-esteem, depressive disorder, oppositional behavior, school failure, risk-taking behavior, or family discord.

What can Parents do?

If your son or daughter is identified as having ADHD:

<u>Be engaged:</u> Learn whatever you can about ADHD. Follow the procedure your child's doctor suggests. Keep all recommended sessions for therapy.

<u>Give medicines safely:</u> If your son or daughter is taking ADHD medication, always give drugs at the suggested time and dosage. Keep medication in a safe place.

<u>Work with your son or daughter's school:</u> Ask educators if your son or daughter must have an Individualized Education Programme (IEP). Meet often with instructors to discover how your son or daughter is doing. Interact to help your son or daughter do well.

<u>Mother or father with purpose and warmness</u>: Learn what parenting methods are best for a child with ADHD and which will make ADHD worse. Chat openly and supportively about ADHD with your son or daughter. *Focus on your son or daughter's advantages and positive characteristics.*

Connect with others for support and awareness. Sign up for a support business for ADHD to get improvements in treatment and other information.

Help your child understand ADHD, use educators, and caregivers, and keep an eye on what helps your child.

What can cause ADHD?

It isn't clear what can cause the brain's distinctions of ADHD. There's definite proof that ADHD is mainly inherited. Many kids who have ADHD have a mother or father or relatives with it.

ADHD is not caused by too much playtime, poor parenting, or overeating glucose.

ADHD can improve when kids get treatment, eat healthy food, get enough rest and exercise, and also have supportive parents who learn how to react to ADHD.

Chapter 3

14 Signs of Attention Deficit Hyperactivity Disorder (ADHD)

What's ADHD?

Attention deficit hyperactivity disorder (ADHD) is an organic neurodevelopmental disorder that makes a difference in your child's success in school, as well as their human relationships. The symptoms of ADHD vary and are occasionally difficult to identify.

Lots of the personal symptoms of ADHD should be expected for just about any child to see. So, to produce an analysis of ADHD, your child's doctor should evaluate your son or daughter using several requirements.

ADHD is normally diagnosed in children by enough time they're teens, with the average age of medical diagnosis being seven years old. Teenagers exhibiting symptoms may have ADHD, but they've often shown rather sophisticated symptoms early in life.

14 Common Signs of ADHD in Children

1. Self-focused behavior

A common sign of ADHD is exactly what appears like an inability to identify other people's desires and needs. This can lead to another two signals: *interrupting and trouble waiting around for their turn.*

2. Interrupting

Self-focused behavior could cause a kid with ADHD to interrupt others while they're talking or butt into conversations or games they're not part of.

3. **Trouble waiting around their turn**

Kids with ADHD may have difficulty waiting around for their turn during classroom activities or when doing things with other children.

4. **Emotional turmoil**

A kid with ADHD may have trouble keeping their feelings in check. They could have outbursts of anger at unacceptable times. Youngsters may have temper tantrums.

5. **Fidgetiness**

Children with ADHD often can't sit still. They could try to get right up and run around, fidget, or squirm in their seats when compelled to relax.

6. **Problems playing quietly**

Fidgetiness makes it problematic for kids with ADHD to try out quietly or engage calmly in leisure activities.

7. **Unfinished tasks**

A kid with ADHD may show interest in a large number of different things. However, they may have problems finishing them. For instance, they could start projects, tasks, or research, but move to the next thing that catches their interest before completing.

8. **Insufficient focus**

A kid with ADHD may have trouble paying attention, even though someone is speaking right to them. They'll say they noticed you; however they won't have the ability to repeat back what you merely said.

9. **Avoidance of duties needing expanded mental effort**

This same insufficient focus can result in a child to avoid activities that require a sustained mental effort, such as attention in class or doing homework.

10. **Mistakes**

Children with ADHD can have trouble pursuing instructions that require planning or performing a plan. This may then lead to careless errors, but it doesn't indicate laziness or too little intelligence.

11. **Daydreaming**

Children with ADHD aren't always noisy and loud. Another indication of ADHD has been quieter and less included than other kids. A kid with ADHD may stare into space, daydream, and disregard what's happening around them.

Get Answers from a health care provider in minutes, anytime.

12. **Trouble getting organized**

A kid with ADHD may have difficulty monitoring tasks and activities. This might cause problems at school, as they will get it hard to prioritize research, school tasks, and other projects.

13. **Forgetfulness**

Kids with ADHD may be forgetful in day to day activities. They could forget to do tasks or their research. They could also lose things often, such as playthings.

14. **Symptoms in multiple settings**

A kid with ADHD will show signs of the problem in several sets. For example, they could show insufficient concentration both in school and at home.

Way Forward

All children will exhibit a few of these behaviors sooner or later. Daydreaming, fidgeting, and prolonged interruptions are common behaviors in children. However, you should start taking into consideration the next steps if:

✓ your son or daughter regularly displays signs of ADHD.

This behavior has effects on their success in school and resulting in negative interactions using their peers.

ADHD is treatable. If your son or daughter is identified as having ADHD, review all the treatment plans. Then, set up a periodic to talk with a health care provider or psychologist to look for the best plan of action.

Signs of ADHD

Young man daydreaming in course; it isn't that children

with ADHD can't give attention when they're doing things, they enjoy hearing about subjects they're interested in and have no trouble entering and staying on the task; but when the duty is repeated or annoying, they quickly tune out.

Staying on the right track is another universal problem. Children with ADHD often jump from task to task without completing some of them or miss the necessary steps. Arranging their schoolwork and their time is harder for them than it is for some children. Kids with ADHD likewise have trouble focusing if things are happening around them; they often need a quiet environment to be able to stay concentrated.

Symptoms of Inattention in Children

✓ Have trouble staying focused; is easily distracted

or gets uninterested in an activity before it's completed.

✓ Appears never to listen when spoken to.

✓ Has difficulty keeping in mind things and subsequent instructions; doesn't focus on details or makes careless mistakes.

✓ Has trouble staying organized, preparing in advance, and finishing projects.

✓ Frequently loses or misplaces homework, books, toys, or other items.

Hyperactivity Signs or Symptoms of ADHD

The most apparent sign of ADHD is hyperactivity. Even though many children usually are quite energetic, kids with hyperactive symptoms of attention deficit disorder are always moving. *They could make an effort to do several things at once, jumping around in one activity to another. Even when pressured to sit down still, which may be very difficult to them, their feet are tapping, their lower leg is shaking, or their fingertips are drumming.*

Symptoms of hyperactivity in children

✓ Constantly fidgets and squirms.

✓ Has difficulty seated still, taking part in things quietly or relaxing?

✓ Works around constantly often work or climb inappropriately.

✓ Talks excessively.

✓ May have an instant temper or "brief fuse."

Impulsive Signs or Symptoms of ADHD

The impulsivity of children with ADHD can cause issues with self-control. Because they censor themselves significantly less than other kids do, they'll interrupt interactions, invade other people's space, ask irrelevant questions in course, make tactless observations, and have excessively personal questions. Instructions like *"Show* patience" and *"Just wait around for a time"* are doubly hard for children with ADHD to check out because they are for other children.

Children with impulsive signs or symptoms of ADHD *also tend to be moody and also to overreact emotionally. Because of this, others may begin to view the kid as disrespectful, strange, or needy.*

Symptoms of impulsivity in children

✓ Functions without thinking.

✓ Guesses, rather than taking time to resolve a problem or blurts out answers in course without waiting around to be called on or hear the complete question.

✓ Intrudes on other people's discussions or games.

✓ Often interrupts others; says the incorrect thing at the wrong time.

✓ Failure to keep powerful feelings in check, leading to angry outbursts or temper tantrums.

Chapter 4

Effect of ADHD in Children

ADHD has nothing in connection with intelligence or skill. What's more, kids with attention deficit disorder often demonstrate the following positive characteristics:

- **Creativeness:** Children who have ADHD can be marvelously creative and imaginative. *The kids who daydream and have ten different thoughts simultaneously may become a grasp problem solver, a fountain of ideas, or an inventive designer.* Children with ADHD may be easily distracted, but sometimes they see what others don't see.

- **Versatility:** Because children with ADHD look at a lot of options simultaneously, they don't become accustomed to one option in the early stages and are more available to different ideas.

- **Excitement and spontaneity:** Children with ADHD are rarely bored! They're thinking about a lot of various things and have energetic personalities. In a nutshell, if they're not exasperating you (or even when they may be), they're lots of fun to be with.

- **Energy and drive:** When kids with ADHD are motivated, they work or play hard and make an effort to succeed. It actually may be difficult to distract them from an activity that is passionate to them, mainly if the experience is interactive or hands-on.

Could it be ADHD?

A child that has symptoms of inattention, impulsivity, or hyperactivity will not mean that he or she has ADHD. Specific medical ailments, mental disorders, and stressful lifestyle occasions can cause symptoms that appear to be ADHD. Before a precise analysis of ADHD can be produced, you must visit a mental doctor to explore and eliminate the following options:

- ✓ Learning disabilities or issues with reading, writing, creative skills, or vocabulary.

- ✓ Major life events or distressing encounters (e.g. a recently available move, loss of life of someone you care about, bullying, divorce).

- ✓ Psychological disorders including anxiety, depression, and bipolar disorder.

- ✓ Behavioral disorders such as conduct disorder,

reactive attachment disorder, and oppositional defiant disorder.

✓ Medical ailments, including thyroid problems, neurological conditions, epilepsy, and sleep problems.

Chapter 5

ADHD Fail-proof Solution

If your child's symptoms of inattention, hyperactivity, and impulsivity are credited to ADHD, they can cause many problems if they remain untreated. Children who can't concentrate and control themselves may struggle in school, get into regular trouble, and discover it's hard to be friends with others or socialize. These frustrations and concerns can result in low self-esteem as well as friction and stress for your family.

But treatment can make a dramatic difference in your child's symptoms. Using the right support, your son or daughter can get on monitor for success in every region of life. If your son or daughter has challenges with symptoms that appear to be ADHD, don't wait around, seek specialized help. You can treat your child's symptoms of hyperactivity, inattention, and impulsivity with no analysis of attention deficit disorder. Options to begin with include getting the child into *therapy, applying a better exercise and diet plan, and changing the house environment to reduce distractions.*

If you do get an analysis of ADHD, after that, you can use your child's doctor, therapist, and college to produce a personalized treatment solution that meets his/her specific needs. The effective treatment for child years of ADHD requires behavioral therapy, mother or father education and training, interpersonal support, and assistance in school. *Medication could also be used; however, it will never be the only real attention deficit disorder treatment.*

School Methods for Children with ADHD

ADHD certainly gets solved in the form of learning. You can't absorb information or get your projects done if you're playing around the classroom or zoning from what you're said to be reading or hearing.

Think about what the institution establishment requires children to do; *Sit down still; Listen silently; Pay attention*; *Follow instructions; Focus.* These are the things kids with ADHD have trouble doing, not because they aren't prepared, but because their brains won't let them. But that doesn't mean kids with ADHD can't succeed in school.

There are a lot of things both parents and educators can do to help children with ADHD thrive in the class. It begins with analyzing each child's specific weaknesses and talents, then discovering creative approaches for helping the kid focus, stick to task, and figure out how to explore his/her full capability.

Parenting Methods for Helping Children with ADHD

"Mother, if your son or daughter is hyperactive, inattentive, or impulsive, it might take a great deal of energy to get her or him to listen, end an activity, or sit still. The continuous monitoring can be annoying and exhausting. Sometimes you might feel like your son or daughter is operating the show. Still, there are actions you can take to regain control of the problem, while simultaneously assisting your son or daughter make the majority of his/her abilities.

While attention deficit disorder is not triggered by bad parenting, there are parenting strategies that can go quite a distance to improve problem behaviors. Children with ADHD need framework, uniformity, clear communication, rewards, and effects for his/her behavior. *Also, they need plenty of love, support, and encouragement.*

There are a lot of things parents can do to lessen the signs or symptoms of ADHD without sacrificing the natural energy, playfulness, and sense of wonder in the child.

Look after yourself, so you're better in a position to care for your son or daughter. Eat right, exercise, get enough rest, find ways to lessen stress, and seek face-to-face support from relatives and buddies, and your child's doctor and instructors.

Establish structure and stay with it. Help your son or daughter remain concentrated and structured by pursuing daily routines, simplifying your child's routine, and maintaining that your child gets occupied with healthy activities.

Set clear anticipations. Make the guidelines of behavior simple and clarify what will happen when these are obeyed or broken, and continue every time with an incentive or an outcome.

Encourage exercise and sleep. Physical activity enhances focus and promotes brain development. Significantly for children with ADHD, it also leads to increased sleep, which can decrease the symptoms of ADHD.

Help your son or daughter eat right. To control symptoms of ADHD, plan regular healthy foods or snacks every three hours, and scale back on junk and sweet food.

Teach your son or daughter steps to make friends. Help him or her become a much better listener, figure out how to read people's encounters and body gestures, and interact more efficiently with others.

Chapter 6

10 Typical Behaviour in ADHD Kids

Knowing the difference between a standard, antsy 4-year-old, and a person who is hyperactive to the stage where it affects his/her ability to learn is becoming trickier as attention deficit disorders have grown to be more common, concerning recent research.

Attention Deficit Hyperactivity Disorder (ADHD) is the most diagnosed mental health disorder among kids in preschool, which is now within one of each 11 school-age children. But forty percent of most 4-year-olds have an issue with attention. So for parents recognizing which behaviors are an indicator of the disorder, is of paramount importance for getting the correct medical diagnosis and treatment, experts say.

"ADHD has a biological basis that often helps it be a lifelong condition. You want to capture ADHD early since it has such a serious influence on learning and educational development," says **Dr. Tag Mahone**, director of neuropsychology at the Kennedy Krieger Institute in Baltimore.

"Understanding the mind variations that happen in people who have ADHD may help in properly diagnosing and dealing with kids," **Mahone** said. For instance, research shows a brain region called the caudate nuclei is smaller in children with ADHD than in other children. The spot is accountable for skills and cognitive control.

But there are noticeable symptoms of ADHD to view for too. Mahone recommended that parents seek advice from their physician if indeed they see these behaviors in their 3- or 4-years-old:

- ✓ *Regular climbing* - even though instructed never to do so.

- ✓ Continuous motion, such as shaking a leg constantly, the shortcoming to sit down without squirming, or restless foot, accompanied by regular needs to get right up and maneuver around.

- ✓ Working and moving so quickly, it leads to severe damage, such as stitches, even after having been informed to stop.

- ✓ An inability to relate peacefully with others, and the casual show of an even of aggression that will require removing the kid from a predicament.

- ✓ Being louder and noisier than fellow playmates.

- ✓ Often befriending strangers with little extreme caution.

- ✓ Displaying unusually low dread in situations that may lead the kid into danger.

- ✓ The inability to concentrate for lots of minutes without shedding interest.

- ✓ Refusal to take part in an activity that will require the child's attention for more than a minute or two.

Chapter 7

Natural Treatments for ADHD

Natural Treatments for ADHD

Attention deficit hyperactivity disorder (ADHD) and Attention deficit disorder (ADD) are neurological and behavior-related conditions that cause difficulty in concentrating, impulsiveness and excessive energy.

People with ADHD symptoms not just have challenges concentrating but have painful sitting still. People that have ADHD are usually more disruptive than people with ADD.

ADHD often comes with an onset age group of seven, but this disorder can continue through teenage years and well into adulthood. It's approximated that ADHD affects 9% of American children between the ages range of 13 and 18 and over 4% of adults.

Based on the NIH's Countrywide Institute of Mental Health, "the number of children being identified as having ADHD is increasing, but it is unclear why." Most doctors and research indicate the upsurge in ADHD is straight from the food that children eat, the way they sleep and even the way they breathe.

Recent research shows that sleep deprivation, circadian rhythm disturbances and sleep-disordered breathing (including mouth area breathing) can lead to the induction of ADHD-like symptoms.

Researchers claim that the long-term effects of ADHD include dire psychological, educational, and psychiatric outcomes. Early analysis and intervention are essential factors in avoiding the debilitating implications of this condition.

Root Factors behind ADD/ADHD

According to many international studies, ADHD has a genetic link. Furthermore, there are environmental factors and diet concerns that lots of researchers believe boost the risk and perhaps, worsens the symptoms.

Processed sugar, artificial sweeteners, a chemical substance in food additives, dietary deficiencies, preservatives and food allergies are factors behind ADD/ADHD.

In children, an incomplete cause relates to too little interest or forcing children to learn in a way that they are not interested in. Some children learn better by watching or doing (kinesthetic), rather than by hearing.

Symptoms of ADD/ADHD

The severe nature of symptoms may differ significantly from individual to individual, depending on environment, diet and other factors.

Children may display a number of the following symptoms of ADHD/ADD

Difficulty in concentrating and diminished focus

- Easily distracted.

- Easily bored.

- Difficulty organizing or completing tasks.

- Susceptible to losing things.

- Doesn't listen.

- Difficulty in following instructions.

- Fidgety behavior, squirming.

- Extreme difficulty being still and quiet.

- Impatience.

Adults may show a number of the following symptoms of ADD/ADHD.

- Difficulty centering and focusing on a task, job, or conversation.

- Overwhelming psychological and physical restlessness.

- Regular mood swings.

- Susceptible to anger and a hot temper.

- Disorganized.

- Low tolerance of individuals, situations, and surroundings.

- Unstable relationships.

- Increased risk for addiction.

The most frequent treatment of ADD/ADHD today is using medications such as **Ritalin and Adderall,** both of which have been associated with suicidal thoughts and personality changes. ***Ritalin*** *is a central nervous system stimulant, that can cause nervousness, agitation, panic, insomnia, vomiting, an elevated heartbeat, increased blood circulation pressure and even psychosis.*

Adderall *can be an amphetamine that is highly addictive with prolonged use. Unwanted effects include tremors, hallucinations, muscle twitches, high blood circulation pressure, fast or abnormal heartbeats, and extreme disposition swings.*

With these side effects, it is simple to understand why

more people would like effective natural treatments for ADHD. The glad tidings are there are natural treatments for ADD/ADHD that are both effective and without the frightening side effects of prescription medications, which includes pursuing an ADHD diet.

ADHD Foods to Avoid

- *Sugar:* This is the main trigger for some children, plus some adults with ADHD. Avoid any types of refined sugar including chocolate, desserts, soda pop or fruit drinks.

- *Gluten:* Some researchers and parents record worsening behavior when the youngster eats gluten, which might indicate sensitivity to the protein within wheat. Avoid all foodstuffs made with whole wheat such as bread, pasta and whole wheat cereal. Search for gluten-free or even grain-free alternatives.

- *Conventional Dairy products:* Most cow milk dairy contains A1 casein that can trigger an identical response as gluten and, for that reason, should be eliminated. If severe symptoms occur after eating dairy products, discontinue use. Goat's dairy, however, will not contain the proteins and is a much better option for some with ADD/ADHD.

- *Food Color and Dyes:* Children with ADHD can be private to several food dyes and colorings; therefore all processed food items should be avoided. Colorings and dyes come in almost every commercially prepared food. Food dyes are available in sports drinks, chocolate, wedding cake mixes, chewable vitamin supplements and even toothpaste!

- *Caffeine:* Although some studies show that caffeine can help with some ADHD symptoms, it pays to reduce or avoid caffeine, as these studies have never been validated. Furthermore, the side effects of caffeine, including lack of reduction, anxiousness, and nervousness, can donate to the symptoms of ADD/ADHD.

- MSG and HVP - Both of these additives are thought to lower dopamine levels in both children and adults. Dopamine is from the brain's pleasure and prize systems. For people battling with ADD/ADHD, well-balanced degrees of dopamine is crucial.

- *Nitrites:* Commonly with lunchmeat, canned foods, and many processed food items, nitrites are associated with a rise of years as a child type one diabetes, and certain types of malignancy and IBS. Furthermore, it can cause a fast heartbeat, difficulty inhaling and exhaling, and restlessness that aggravate ADHD symptoms.

- *Artificial Sweeteners*: Artificial sweeteners are just harmful to your health, but also for those coping with ADHD; the medial side effects can be damaging. Artificial sweeteners create biochemical changes in the torso, a few of which could harm cognitive function and psychological balance.

- *Soy:* Soy is a typical food allergen and can disrupt hormones that cause ADHD.

- *Personal Food Sensitivities/Things that trigger allergies:* Get rid of the top seven allergens, including soy, wheat, and conventional dairy mentioned previously, as well as peanuts, tree nuts, eggs and shellfish. Furthermore, eliminate any foods or drinks that are personal things that trigger allergies. This may include papaya, avocados, bananas and kiwis (for people that have latex allergies) and coriander, caraway or fennel (all from the same family), and chocolates.

Top 5 Natural Supplements for ADHD

I believe that incorporating new foods into the diet alongside eliminating dangerous foods are essential; these five supplements represent vital natural treatments for ADHD.

1. *Fish Essential oil (Omega-3) (1,000 milligrams daily)*

Omega 3 supplements have proven to be beneficial to ADHD patients, as the EPA/DHA in seafood oil is crucial for brain function and is anti-inflammatory. Supplementation has proven to lessen symptoms and improve learning.

2. *B-Complex (50 milligrams daily)*

Children with ADHD might need more *B-vitamins* to assist with the forming of serotonin, especially Vitamin B6.

3. *Multi-Mineral Product (including zinc, magnesium and calcium mineral)*

I would recommend that a person with ADHD take 500 milligrams of calcium mineral, 250 milligrams of magnesium and 5 milligrams double zinc daily. All are likely involved in calming the nervous system and insufficiency may exacerbate symptoms.

4. *Probiotic (25-50 billion models daily)*

ADHD may be linked to digestive issues, therefore going for a good quality probiotic daily can help maintain intestinal health.

5. *GABA (250 milligrams double daily)*

A relaxing amino acidity, ask your physician before taking GABA, as it could interact with other medications.

Other rewarding supplements are;

Rhodiola Rosea has shown effectiveness in enhancing the attention of both adults and children. It functions by increasing the level of sensitivity in the neurological and nervous system that produce serotonin and dopamine, that are both needed for effective ADHD indicator control.

Essential Oils for ADHD

According to a report conducted by *Dr. Terry Friedmann*, essential natural oils of vetiver and cedarwood are incredibly useful in enhancing focus and soothing down children with ADHD.

For memory space and focus, *rosemary and peppermint oils* have proven to boost alertness while improving memory.

For a relaxing impact, *Ylang and lavender* works, while *frankincense* brings psychological wellness, clearness and heightened cognitive function.

Top Foods for ADHD

- *Additive-free, Unprocessed Foods:* Because of the harmful nature of food additives, it is advisable to eat unprocessed, fresh foods. Additives, including artificial sweeteners, preservatives, and colorings that exist within processed food items, maybe especially detrimental for people that have ADD/ADHD.

- *Foods Saturated in B-Vitamins* - B vitamin supplements help maintain a wholesome nervous system. Be sure to include organic animal products and a lot of green leafy vegetables in what you eat. Based on the University of Maryland INFIRMARY, Vitamin B-6 is necessary for your body and uses essential brain chemicals including *serotonin, dopamine and norepinephrine*. One preliminary research has discovered that B-6 is somewhat far better than Ritalin in enhancing behavior! Include wild tuna, bananas, crazy salmon, grass-fed meat and other foodstuffs rich in supplement B-6 for the improvement of ADHD.

- *Chicken:* Tryptophan can be an essential amino acid that helps your body to synthesize proteins and assist in the creation of serotonin. Serotonin takes on significant functions in sleep, swelling, emotional moods plus much more. In lots of individuals experiencing ADD/ADHD, imbalances in serotonin levels have been indicated based on the College or university of Michigan Health System. Serotonin relates to impulse control and hostility, two of the symptoms of ADD/ADHD.

- **_Eat Breakfast:_** For a lot and especially people that have ADHD, breakfast helps your body properly regulate bloodstream sugars and stabilize hormone fluctuations. Eat a breakfast that has at least 20 grams of proteins. Try my Thin Mint Proteins Smoothie that has 20 grams of proteins; it is a delicious and filling up way to "break the fast."

- **_Wild-Caught Salmon:_** It's not only wealthy with vitamin B-6, but it's also filled with omega 3 essential fatty acids. Based on the School of Maryland INFIRMARY, a scientific trial indicated that lower degrees of omega-3 essential fatty acids acquired more learning and behavioral problems (like those associated with ADHD) than kids with reasonable degrees of omega. Individuals, including children, should consume outrageous salmon at least two times per week.

Changes in Lifestyle for Adults with ADHD

Create an Organizational System that works for you - There is undoubtedly no one firm solution that works for everybody. Find the method that is most effective for you. A straightforward pen and paper checklist may be what some need, while some will need a far more specialized technique that could include establishing automated reminders, prioritizing duties and more.

- *Use Technology in your favor:* There are several apps designed for smartphones and tablets for efficiency. These tools can enable you to plan and prioritize tasks. Furthermore, consider noise-canceling headphones to help push away the distractions in your house or office.

- *Exercise:* Regular physical activity not only helps build muscles and bone but helps to relieve stress. Furthermore, to your regular physical exercise, try something that engages your "fun" gene too. Dance, fighting techniques, playing rugby or volleyball, are great ways to burn off calories, balance hormones and reduce stress.

- *Get more sleep*: Recent research demonstrates sleep deprivation, and circadian tempo disturbances are from the induction of ADHD symptoms. For adults fighting a sleep problem, melatonin foods and supplements, light therapy and neurofeedback therapy can help to ease

ADHD symptoms. Also, sticking with a wholesome, well-balanced diet, getting daily exercise and sleep techniques can enable you to get the others you need. If you don't have a sleep problem, but need to improve your sleep practices, focus on creating regular bedtimes that enable at least seven hours of rest per night time and switch off devices forty-five (45) minutes before sleep.

The diet changes, supplements, and recommended changes in lifestyle above can help you conquer ADD/ADHD. The solutions above are similarly effective for children and adults as well.

For many individuals, removing the ADD/ADHD trigger foods and updating them with well-balanced meals that naturally battle ADD/ADHD will significantly help manage this common neurological and behavioral disorder. Keep in mind, detoxing from many years of chemicals and processed foods take time. Stay with this program above and kick ADD/ADHD once and for all!

Change in Lifestyle for Kids with ADHD

The task for the parents of a kid with ADD/ADHD isn't just to find a highly effective natural treatment for ADHD and ADD, but also to produce a host that supports their creativeness and spurs learning. Below are a few lifestyle changes that might help.

- *Show Devotion (and have for this):* Children coping with ADHD need reassurance they aren't a needy child. If you only react to the negative behaviors, it can result in more negative reactions. Find ways to get along with your son or daughter while keeping them in charge of their actions. Keep in mind; these are more than merely the behaviors of ADHD. Provide them with the opportunity to "WOW" you.

- ***Provide Opportunities for Success***: A kid knows if you are genuinely thrilled and happy on their behalf. Supply them with opportunities where they can be successful. Engage them in creative activities such as painting and sketching. Many top artwork contests in the world have "quick sketch" tournaments that force performers to provide their most excellent work in thirty to forty minutes. Celebrate your child's concentrate and creative soul in these kinds of challenges.

- *Regular exercise & outdoor playtime:* For children with ADHD, burning up some of the surplus energy of your day can help balance hormone levels and offer your son or daughter with the inspiration for healthy bones and muscles.

- Develop a Child-Friendly Organizational System - Find the techniques of corporation that work best for your son or daughter. This may add a notebook with a checklist of daily "to-dos," a graph on the wall structure, or reminders on their smartphones or tablets. Teach them how to prioritize tasks, including school work, home tasks, exercise and fun activities.

- *Teach your son or daughter to make:* Since ADD/ADHD is from the foods consumed and has a genetic link, your son or daughter must learn what foods cause ADD/ADHD and those could cure it. Spend time with your son or daughter discovering exciting ways to prepare wild seafood, grass-fed meat, free-range chicken and fruits and vegetables. Engage them in the menu planning and cooking food process, and the eating changes suggested above will be significantly simpler to implement.

- ***Establish healthy sleep patterns:*** According to an analysis posted in Clinical Psychopharmacology and Neuroscience, sleep deprivation and disturbances to your circadian can donate to the onset or intensity of ADHD symptoms. Plus, experts explain that the long-term implications of sleep issues in people with ADHD include weight problems, poor educational performance and disrupted parent-child relationships. If your son or daughter is fighting a sleep problem or always awake in the middle of the night time, consider natural interventions such as melatonin, light therapy and sleep techniques. It's also essential to determine a night regular that involves sticking with the same bedtime and wake-up time every day.

- *Avoid Mouth Deep breathing:* Research from Japan implies that people who habitually breathe through the mouth area are much more likely than those who breathe through the nose to have ADHD and have sleep problems. This is credited to a notable difference in air load in mind, which can adversely affect brain function in both children and adults. Mouth area breathing causes an elevated air weight to the prefrontal cortex, therefore causing central exhaustion and sleep disruptions.

Why would children inhale through their mouths rather than their noses? The root cause of the mouth area inhaling and exhaling is obstructed nasal airways. To avoid mouth area breathing, you may use sinus dilators that help decrease airflow level of resistance, or your son or daughter can wear a nose and mouth mask during the night that's called constant positive air pressure therapy (CPAP). Speak to your child's pediatrician about these options.

www.ingramcontent.com/pod-product-compliance
Lightning Source LLC
Chambersburg PA
CBHW060346050426
42336CB00050B/2141